Dedicated to Conor and Margaret, who inspired this story,

and to their parents, Abby and Chrys,

whose photographs helped me create the pictures.

My Sister Came Early

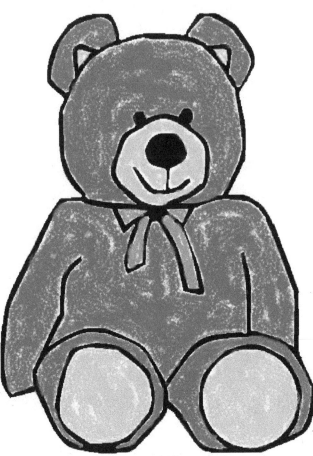

A coloring
book for a kid
with a premature
baby sister.

By S.E. Burr

I have a baby sister.
She is very, very small.

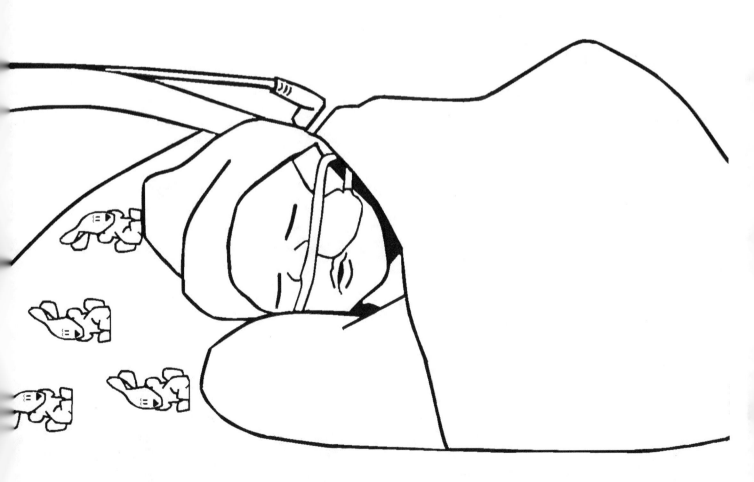

I am her older sibling.

I am big, and strong, and tall.

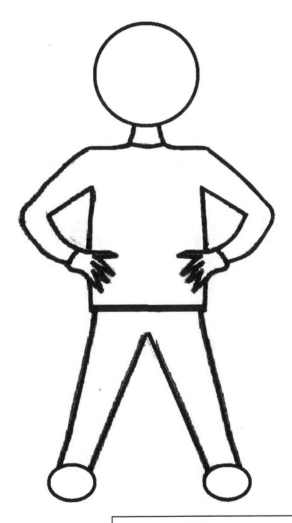

This is you! What does your hair look like? What color are your eyes? What kind of clothes do you like to wear? Draw yourself!

She has itty-bitty fingers
and teeny-weeny toes.

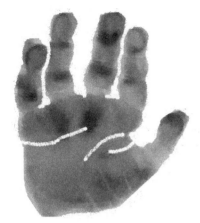
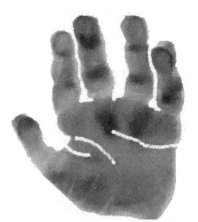
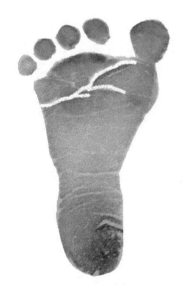
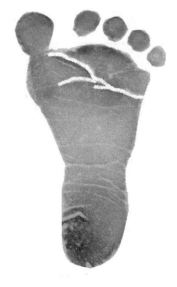

All of her is tiny,

from her feet up to her nose.

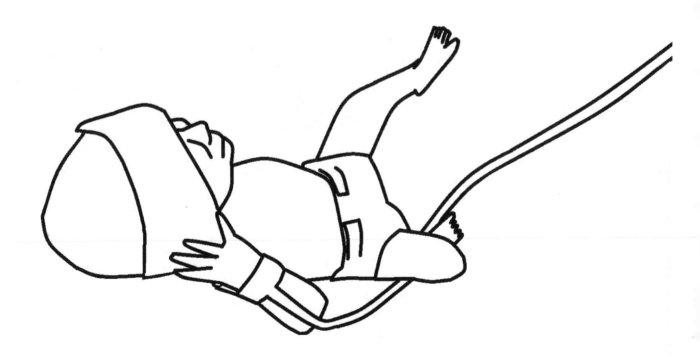

She was in my mommy's belly
but sadly, she couldn't stay.

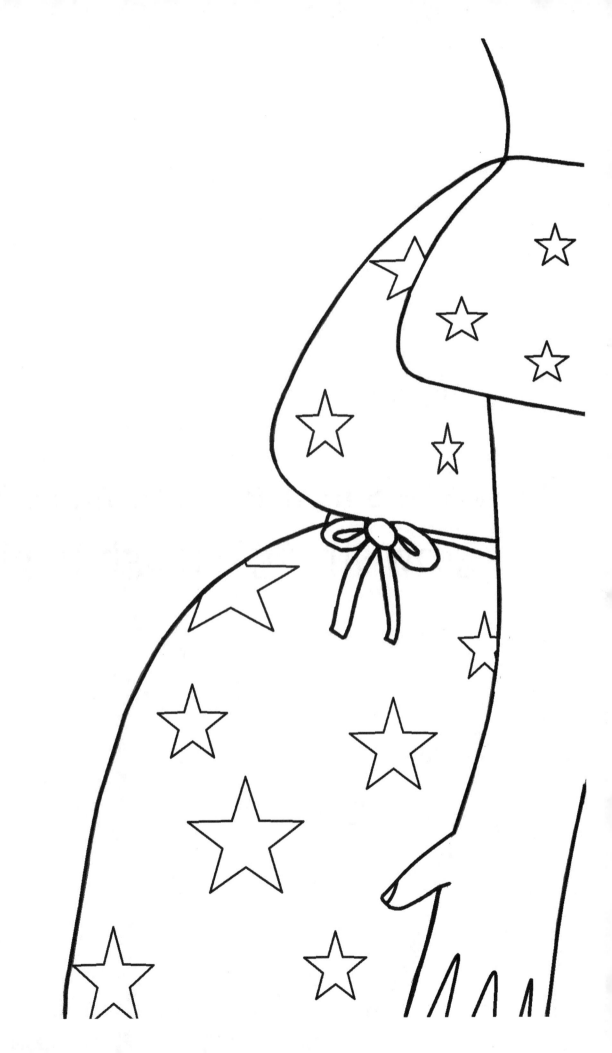

Now she's in the hospital, so she can grow strong enough to play.

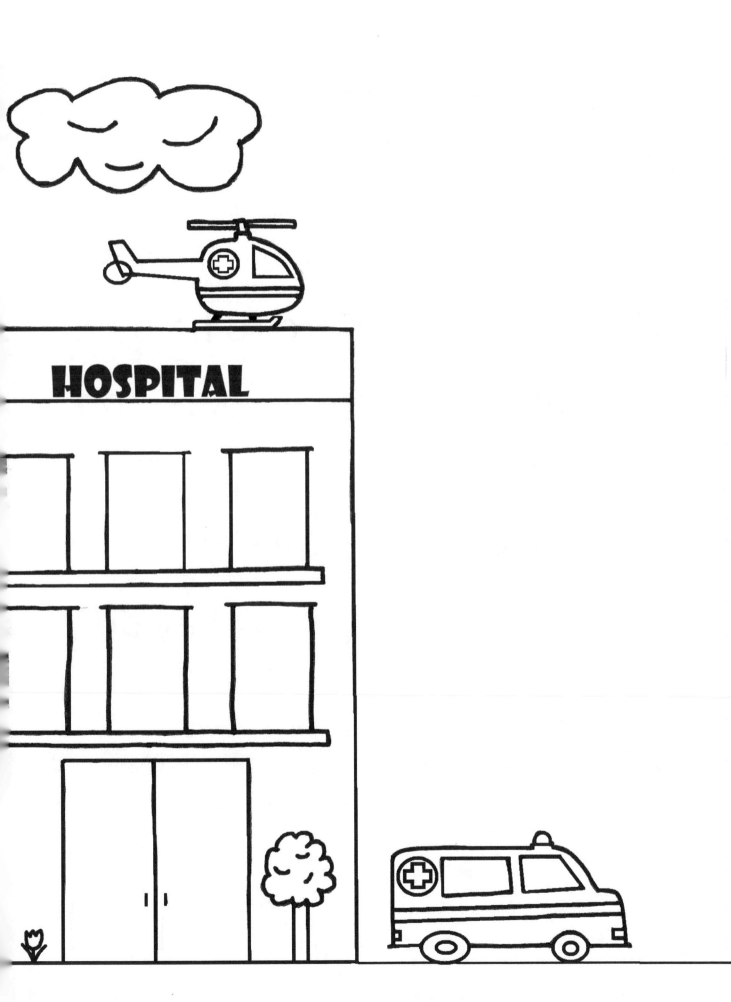

The nurses are there to help her.

The machines are helpers, too.

Listen for a minute,

and I'll tell you what they do.

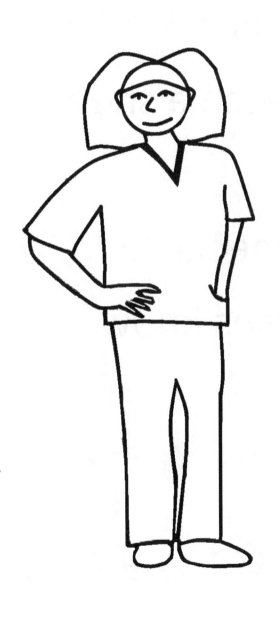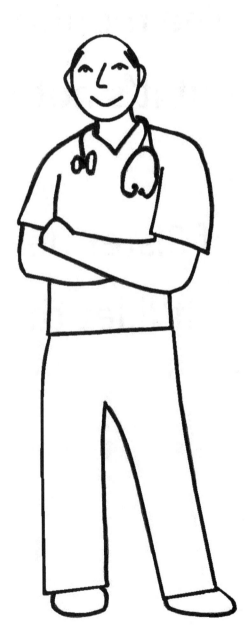

The monitor looks like a TV,
but it's not to watch a show.

If Sister needs special help,
it'll let the nurses know.

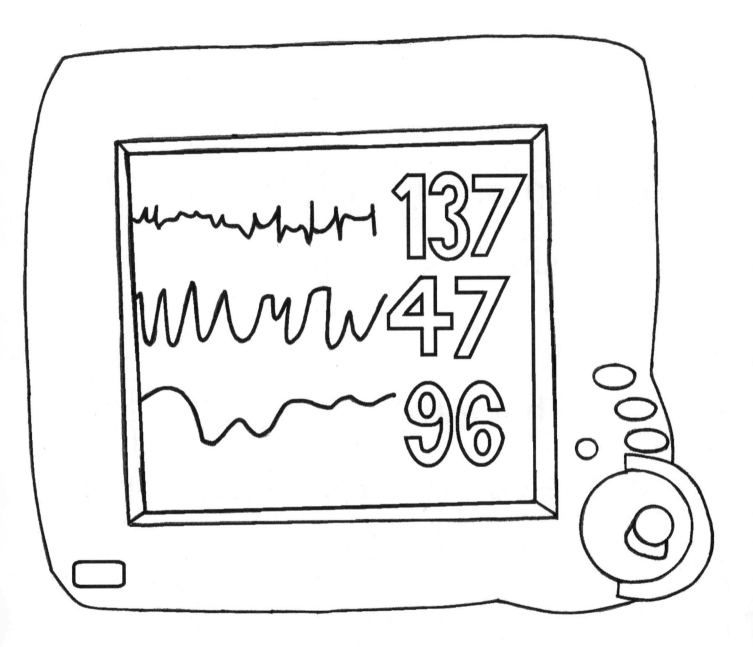

To keep my sister safe and warm,
she has a special bed.

I have to speak quietly
so she can rest her sleepy head.

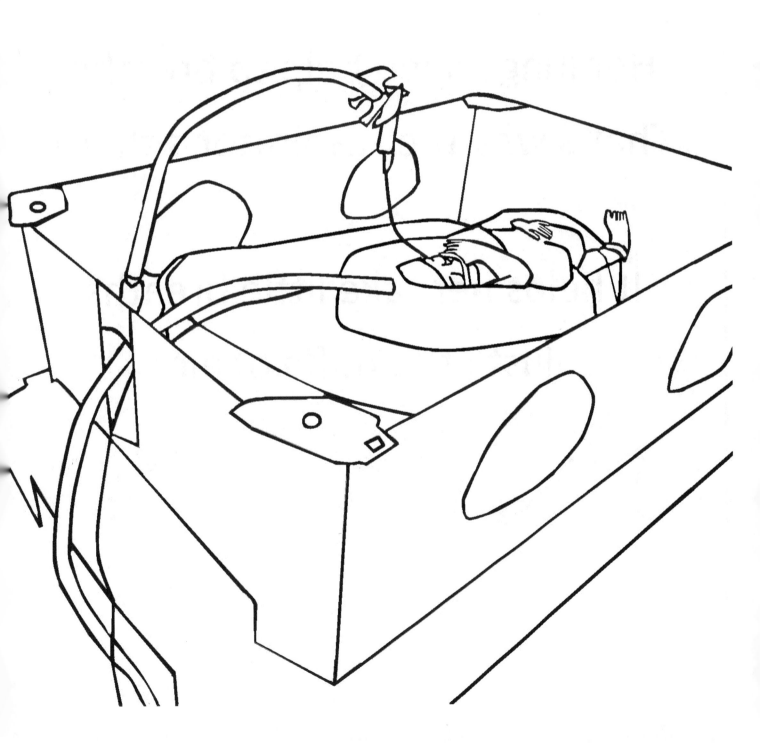

Her lungs need help to breathe.
That's why the respirator's there.

It helps her take little breaths,
just little puffs of air.

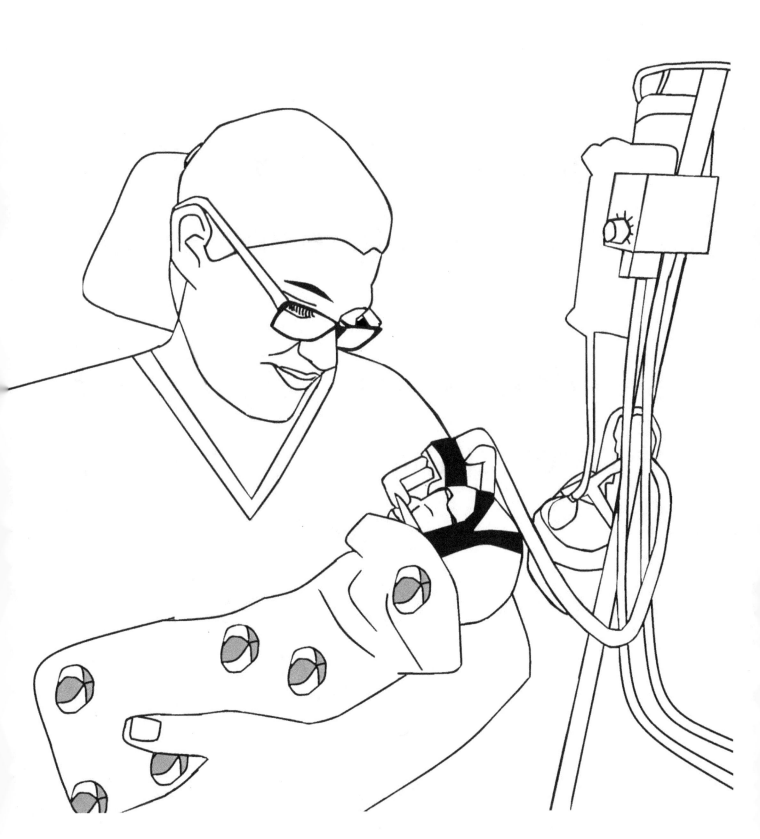

Another helper is called Bili.
He shines so blue and bright.

Sister's eyes wear special glasses
to protect them from the light.

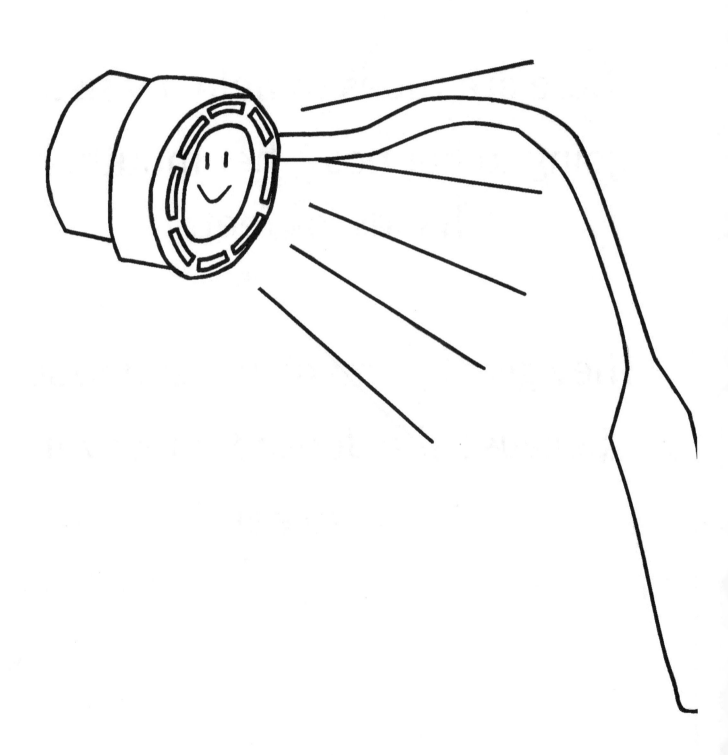

There are tubes to help my sister going to her nose, her mouth, her hands, or feet.

They give her medicine and food, because she doesn't know yet how to eat.

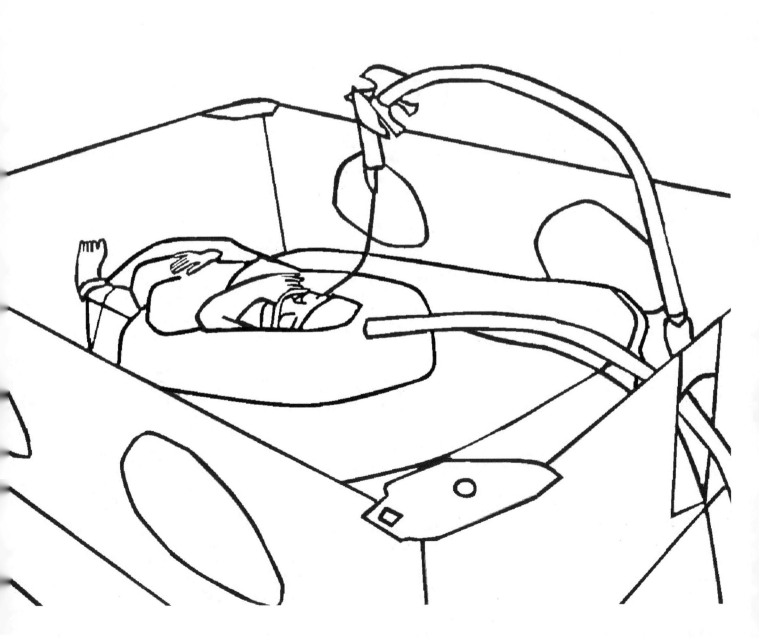

My sister's trying to grow healthy
so her NICU stay can be done.

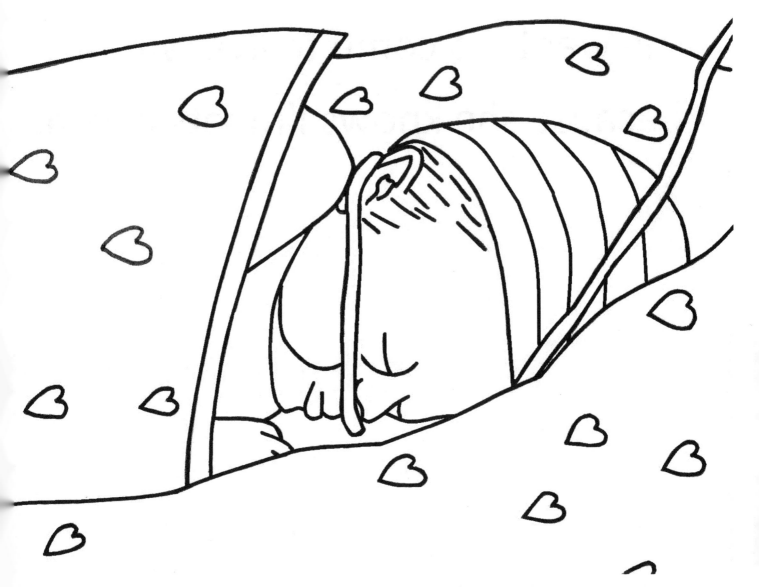

She wants to come to live with me,
because she knows I'm lots of fun.

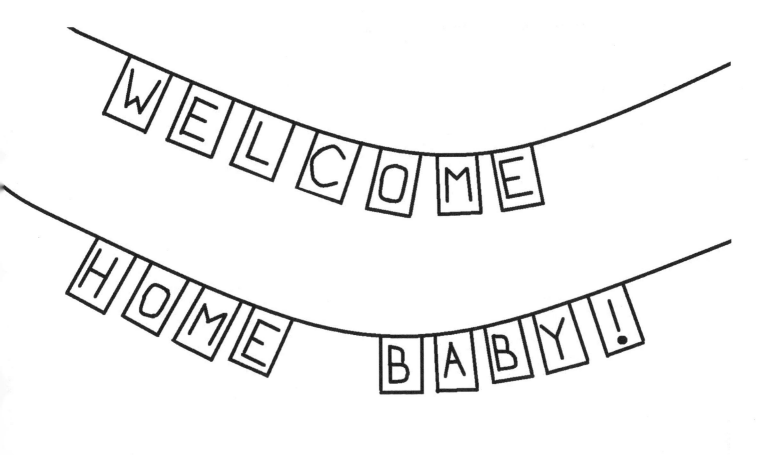

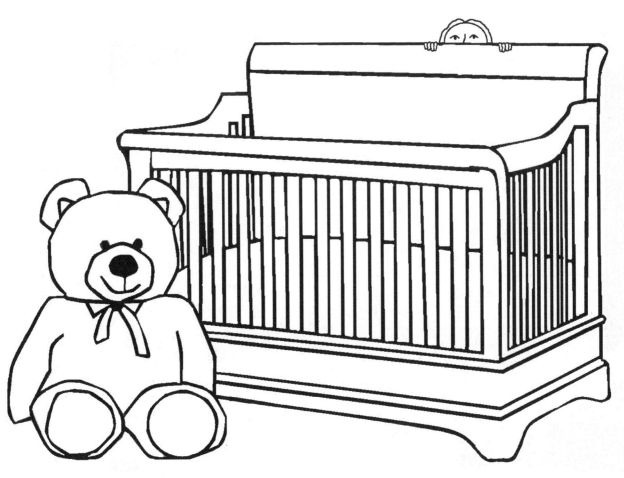

Printed in the USA
CPSIA information can be obtained
at www.ICGtesting.com
LVHW081158141223
766279LV00016B/658